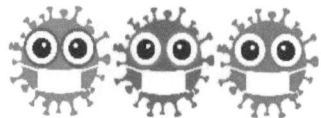

Renate & Uwe H. Sültz
Bücher von A bis Z

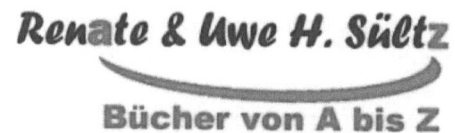

CORONA CONTACT DIARY

AF175256

My name

address

Telephone cell phone email address

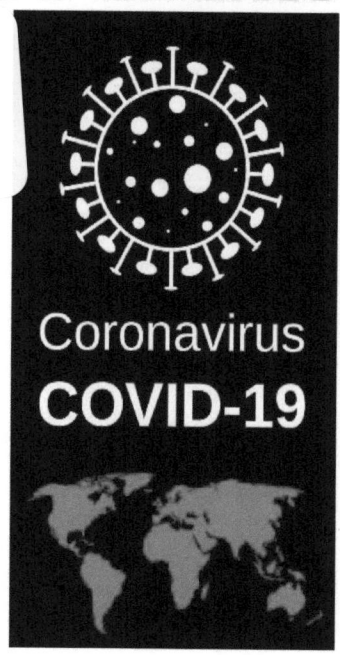

Coronavirus
COVID-19

BoD - Books on Demand
Norderstedt 2020

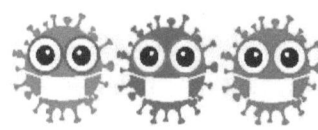

Bibliografische Information durch die Deutsche Nationalbibliothek
Die Deutsche Nationalbibliothek verzeichnet diese Publikation in der
Deutschen Nationalbibliografie; detaillierte bibliografische Daten
sind im Internet über http://dnb.dnb.de abrufbar.

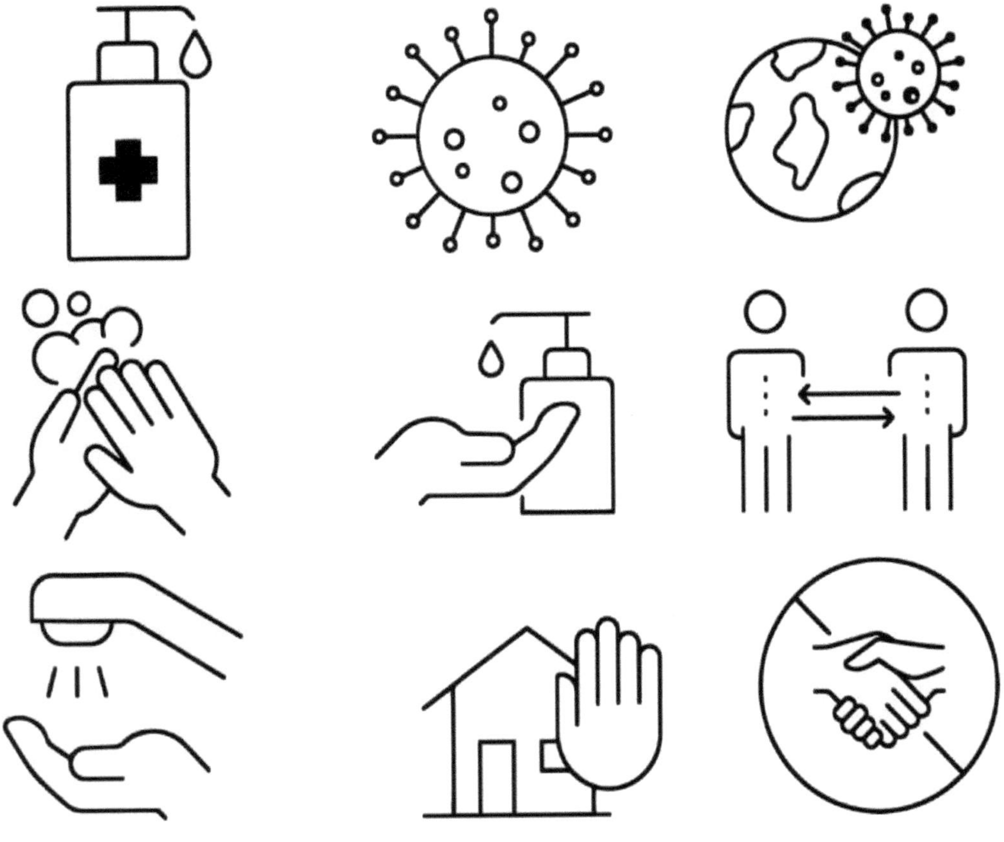

© 2020 Renate & Uwe H. Sültz
Herstellung und Verlag:
BoD – Books on Demand, Norderstedt
ISBN   9-78375-2-64412-8

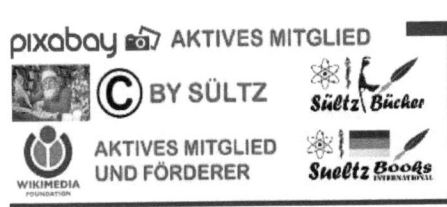

DATE	PLACE	TIME	REASON FOR THE MEETING	

MOUTH AND NOSE PROTECTION ● INDIVIDUAL ● GROUP ●

CLOSED ROOM ● OUTDOORS ● CLOSE CONTACT ●

CONTACT DETAILS

DATE	PLACE	TIME	REASON FOR THE MEETING	

MOUTH AND NOSE PROTECTION ● INDIVIDUAL ● GROUP ●

CLOSED ROOM ● OUTDOORS ● CLOSE CONTACT ●

CONTACT DETAILS

DATE	PLACE	TIME	REASON FOR THE MEETING	

MOUTH AND NOSE PROTECTION ● INDIVIDUAL ● GROUP ●

CLOSED ROOM ● OUTDOORS ● CLOSE CONTACT ●

CONTACT DETAILS

DATE	PLACE	TIME	REASON FOR THE MEETING	

MOUTH AND NOSE PROTECTION ● INDIVIDUAL ● GROUP ●

CLOSED ROOM ● OUTDOORS ● CLOSE CONTACT ●

CONTACT DETAILS

DATE	PLACE	TIME	REASON FOR THE MEETING	

MOUTH AND NOSE PROTECTION ⬤ INDIVIDUAL ⬤ GROUP ⬤
CLOSED ROOM ⬤ OUTDOORS ⬤ CLOSE CONTACT ⬤

CONTACT DETAILS

DATE	PLACE	TIME	REASON FOR THE MEETING	

MOUTH AND NOSE PROTECTION ⬤ INDIVIDUAL ⬤ GROUP ⬤
CLOSED ROOM ⬤ OUTDOORS ⬤ CLOSE CONTACT ⬤

CONTACT DETAILS

DATE	PLACE	TIME	REASON FOR THE MEETING	

MOUTH AND NOSE PROTECTION ⬤ INDIVIDUAL ⬤ GROUP ⬤
CLOSED ROOM ⬤ OUTDOORS ⬤ CLOSE CONTACT ⬤

CONTACT DETAILS

DATE	PLACE	TIME	REASON FOR THE MEETING	

MOUTH AND NOSE PROTECTION ⬤ INDIVIDUAL ⬤ GROUP ⬤
CLOSED ROOM ⬤ OUTDOORS ⬤ CLOSE CONTACT ⬤

CONTACT DETAILS

DATE	PLACE	TIME	REASON FOR THE MEETING	

MOUTH AND NOSE PROTECTION ⬤ CLOSED ROOM ⬤ INDIVIDUAL ⬤ OUTDOORS ⬤ GROUP ⬤ CLOSE CONTACT ⬤

CONTACT DETAILS

DATE	PLACE	TIME	REASON FOR THE MEETING	

MOUTH AND NOSE PROTECTION ⬤ CLOSED ROOM ⬤ INDIVIDUAL ⬤ OUTDOORS ⬤ GROUP ⬤ CLOSE CONTACT ⬤

CONTACT DETAILS

DATE	PLACE	TIME	REASON FOR THE MEETING	

MOUTH AND NOSE PROTECTION ⬤ CLOSED ROOM ⬤ INDIVIDUAL ⬤ OUTDOORS ⬤ GROUP ⬤ CLOSE CONTACT ⬤

CONTACT DETAILS

DATE	PLACE	TIME	REASON FOR THE MEETING	

MOUTH AND NOSE PROTECTION ⬤ CLOSED ROOM ⬤ INDIVIDUAL ⬤ OUTDOORS ⬤ GROUP ⬤ CLOSE CONTACT ⬤

CONTACT DETAILS

DATE	PLACE	TIME	REASON FOR THE MEETING	

MOUTH AND NOSE PROTECTION ⚪ INDIVIDUAL ⚪ GROUP ⚪

CLOSED ROOM ⚪ OUTDOORS ⚪ CLOSE CONTACT ⚪

CONTACT DETAILS

DATE	PLACE	TIME	REASON FOR THE MEETING	

MOUTH AND NOSE PROTECTION ⚪ INDIVIDUAL ⚪ GROUP ⚪

CLOSED ROOM ⚪ OUTDOORS ⚪ CLOSE CONTACT ⚪

CONTACT DETAILS

DATE	PLACE	TIME	REASON FOR THE MEETING	

MOUTH AND NOSE PROTECTION ⚪ INDIVIDUAL ⚪ GROUP ⚪

CLOSED ROOM ⚪ OUTDOORS ⚪ CLOSE CONTACT ⚪

CONTACT DETAILS

DATE	PLACE	TIME	REASON FOR THE MEETING	

MOUTH AND NOSE PROTECTION ⚪ INDIVIDUAL ⚪ GROUP ⚪

CLOSED ROOM ⚪ OUTDOORS ⚪ CLOSE CONTACT ⚪

CONTACT DETAILS

DATE	PLACE	TIME	REASON FOR THE MEETING	

MOUTH AND NOSE PROTECTION ⬤
CLOSED ROOM ⬤
INDIVIDUAL ⬤
OUTDOORS ⬤
GROUP ⬤
CLOSE CONTACT ⬤

CONTACT DETAILS

DATE	PLACE	TIME	REASON FOR THE MEETING	

MOUTH AND NOSE PROTECTION ⬤
CLOSED ROOM ⬤
INDIVIDUAL ⬤
OUTDOORS ⬤
GROUP ⬤
CLOSE CONTACT ⬤

CONTACT DETAILS

DATE	PLACE	TIME	REASON FOR THE MEETING	

MOUTH AND NOSE PROTECTION ⬤
CLOSED ROOM ⬤
INDIVIDUAL ⬤
OUTDOORS ⬤
GROUP ⬤
CLOSE CONTACT ⬤

CONTACT DETAILS

DATE	PLACE	TIME	REASON FOR THE MEETING	

MOUTH AND NOSE PROTECTION ⬤
CLOSED ROOM ⬤
INDIVIDUAL ⬤
OUTDOORS ⬤
GROUP ⬤
CLOSE CONTACT ⬤

CONTACT DETAILS

DATE	PLACE	TIME	REASON FOR THE MEETING	

MOUTH AND NOSE PROTECTION ⬤   INDIVIDUAL ⬤   GROUP ⬤

CLOSED ROOM ⬤   OUTDOORS ⬤   CLOSE CONTACT ⬤

CONTACT DETAILS

DATE	PLACE	TIME	REASON FOR THE MEETING	

MOUTH AND NOSE PROTECTION ⬤   INDIVIDUAL ⬤   GROUP ⬤

CLOSED ROOM ⬤   OUTDOORS ⬤   CLOSE CONTACT ⬤

CONTACT DETAILS

DATE	PLACE	TIME	REASON FOR THE MEETING	

MOUTH AND NOSE PROTECTION ⬤   INDIVIDUAL ⬤   GROUP ⬤

CLOSED ROOM ⬤   OUTDOORS ⬤   CLOSE CONTACT ⬤

CONTACT DETAILS

DATE	PLACE	TIME	REASON FOR THE MEETING	

MOUTH AND NOSE PROTECTION ⬤   INDIVIDUAL ⬤   GROUP ⬤

CLOSED ROOM ⬤   OUTDOORS ⬤   CLOSE CONTACT ⬤

CONTACT DETAILS

DATE	PLACE	TIME	REASON FOR THE MEETING	

MOUTH AND NOSE PROTECTION ⚪ CLOSED ROOM ⚪   INDIVIDUAL ⚪ GROUP ⚪ OUTDOORS ⚪ CLOSE CONTACT ⚪

CONTACT DETAILS

DATE	PLACE	TIME	REASON FOR THE MEETING	

MOUTH AND NOSE PROTECTION ⚪ CLOSED ROOM ⚪   INDIVIDUAL ⚪ GROUP ⚪ OUTDOORS ⚪ CLOSE CONTACT ⚪

CONTACT DETAILS

DATE	PLACE	TIME	REASON FOR THE MEETING	

MOUTH AND NOSE PROTECTION ⚪ CLOSED ROOM ⚪   INDIVIDUAL ⚪ GROUP ⚪ OUTDOORS ⚪ CLOSE CONTACT ⚪

CONTACT DETAILS

DATE	PLACE	TIME	REASON FOR THE MEETING	

MOUTH AND NOSE PROTECTION ⚪ CLOSED ROOM ⚪   INDIVIDUAL ⚪ GROUP ⚪ OUTDOORS ⚪ CLOSE CONTACT ⚪

CONTACT DETAILS

DATE	PLACE	TIME	REASON FOR THE MEETING	

MOUTH AND NOSE PROTECTION ⬤   INDIVIDUAL ⬤   GROUP ⬤
CLOSED ROOM ⬤   OUTDOORS ⬤   CLOSE CONTACT ⬤

CONTACT DETAILS

DATE	PLACE	TIME	REASON FOR THE MEETING	

MOUTH AND NOSE PROTECTION ⬤   INDIVIDUAL ⬤   GROUP ⬤
CLOSED ROOM ⬤   OUTDOORS ⬤   CLOSE CONTACT ⬤

CONTACT DETAILS

DATE	PLACE	TIME	REASON FOR THE MEETING	

MOUTH AND NOSE PROTECTION ⬤   INDIVIDUAL ⬤   GROUP ⬤
CLOSED ROOM ⬤   OUTDOORS ⬤   CLOSE CONTACT ⬤

CONTACT DETAILS

DATE	PLACE	TIME	REASON FOR THE MEETING	

MOUTH AND NOSE PROTECTION ⬤   INDIVIDUAL ⬤   GROUP ⬤
CLOSED ROOM ⬤   OUTDOORS ⬤   CLOSE CONTACT ⬤

CONTACT DETAILS

DATE	PLACE	TIME	REASON FOR THE MEETING	

MOUTH AND NOSE PROTECTION ○   INDIVIDUAL ○   GROUP ○
CLOSED ROOM ○   OUTDOORS ○   CLOSE CONTACT ○

CONTACT DETAILS

DATE	PLACE	TIME	REASON FOR THE MEETING	

MOUTH AND NOSE PROTECTION ○   INDIVIDUAL ○   GROUP ○
CLOSED ROOM ○   OUTDOORS ○   CLOSE CONTACT ○

CONTACT DETAILS

DATE	PLACE	TIME	REASON FOR THE MEETING	

MOUTH AND NOSE PROTECTION ○   INDIVIDUAL ○   GROUP ○
CLOSED ROOM ○   OUTDOORS ○   CLOSE CONTACT ○

CONTACT DETAILS

DATE	PLACE	TIME	REASON FOR THE MEETING	

MOUTH AND NOSE PROTECTION ○   INDIVIDUAL ○   GROUP ○
CLOSED ROOM ○   OUTDOORS ○   CLOSE CONTACT ○

CONTACT DETAILS

DATE	PLACE	TIME	REASON FOR THE MEETING	

MOUTH AND NOSE PROTECTION ⬤
CLOSED ROOM ⬤

INDIVIDUAL ⬤
OUTDOORS ⬤

GROUP ⬤
CLOSE CONTACT ⬤

CONTACT DETAILS

DATE	PLACE	TIME	REASON FOR THE MEETING	

MOUTH AND NOSE PROTECTION ⬤
CLOSED ROOM ⬤

INDIVIDUAL ⬤
OUTDOORS ⬤

GROUP ⬤
CLOSE CONTACT ⬤

CONTACT DETAILS

DATE	PLACE	TIME	REASON FOR THE MEETING	

MOUTH AND NOSE PROTECTION ⬤
CLOSED ROOM ⬤

INDIVIDUAL ⬤
OUTDOORS ⬤

GROUP ⬤
CLOSE CONTACT ⬤

CONTACT DETAILS

DATE	PLACE	TIME	REASON FOR THE MEETING	

MOUTH AND NOSE PROTECTION ⬤
CLOSED ROOM ⬤

INDIVIDUAL ⬤
OUTDOORS ⬤

GROUP ⬤
CLOSE CONTACT ⬤

CONTACT DETAILS

DATE	PLACE	TIME	REASON FOR THE MEETING	

MOUTH AND NOSE PROTECTION ●   INDIVIDUAL ●   GROUP ●

CLOSED ROOM ●   OUTDOORS ●   CLOSE CONTACT ●

CONTACT DETAILS

DATE	PLACE	TIME	REASON FOR THE MEETING	

MOUTH AND NOSE PROTECTION ●   INDIVIDUAL ●   GROUP ●

CLOSED ROOM ●   OUTDOORS ●   CLOSE CONTACT ●

CONTACT DETAILS

DATE	PLACE	TIME	REASON FOR THE MEETING	

MOUTH AND NOSE PROTECTION ●   INDIVIDUAL ●   GROUP ●

CLOSED ROOM ●   OUTDOORS ●   CLOSE CONTACT ●

CONTACT DETAILS

DATE	PLACE	TIME	REASON FOR THE MEETING	

MOUTH AND NOSE PROTECTION ●   INDIVIDUAL ●   GROUP ●

CLOSED ROOM ●   OUTDOORS ●   CLOSE CONTACT ●

CONTACT DETAILS

DATE	PLACE	TIME	REASON FOR THE MEETING	

MOUTH AND NOSE PROTECTION ⬤   INDIVIDUAL ⬤   GROUP ⬤
CLOSED ROOM ⬤   OUTDOORS ⬤   CLOSE CONTACT ⬤

CONTACT DETAILS

DATE	PLACE	TIME	REASON FOR THE MEETING	

MOUTH AND NOSE PROTECTION ⬤   INDIVIDUAL ⬤   GROUP ⬤
CLOSED ROOM ⬤   OUTDOORS ⬤   CLOSE CONTACT ⬤

CONTACT DETAILS

DATE	PLACE	TIME	REASON FOR THE MEETING	

MOUTH AND NOSE PROTECTION ⬤   INDIVIDUAL ⬤   GROUP ⬤
CLOSED ROOM ⬤   OUTDOORS ⬤   CLOSE CONTACT ⬤

CONTACT DETAILS

DATE	PLACE	TIME	REASON FOR THE MEETING	

MOUTH AND NOSE PROTECTION ⬤   INDIVIDUAL ⬤   GROUP ⬤
CLOSED ROOM ⬤   OUTDOORS ⬤   CLOSE CONTACT ⬤

CONTACT DETAILS

DATE	PLACE	TIME	REASON FOR THE MEETING	

MOUTH AND NOSE PROTECTION ⚪
INDIVIDUAL ⚪
GROUP ⚪
CLOSED ROOM ⚪
OUTDOORS ⚪
CLOSE CONTACT ⚪

CONTACT DETAILS

DATE	PLACE	TIME	REASON FOR THE MEETING	

MOUTH AND NOSE PROTECTION ⚪
INDIVIDUAL ⚪
GROUP ⚪
CLOSED ROOM ⚪
OUTDOORS ⚪
CLOSE CONTACT ⚪

CONTACT DETAILS

DATE	PLACE	TIME	REASON FOR THE MEETING	

MOUTH AND NOSE PROTECTION ⚪
INDIVIDUAL ⚪
GROUP ⚪
CLOSED ROOM ⚪
OUTDOORS ⚪
CLOSE CONTACT ⚪

CONTACT DETAILS

DATE	PLACE	TIME	REASON FOR THE MEETING	

MOUTH AND NOSE PROTECTION ⚪
INDIVIDUAL ⚪
GROUP ⚪
CLOSED ROOM ⚪
OUTDOORS ⚪
CLOSE CONTACT ⚪

CONTACT DETAILS

DATE	PLACE	TIME	REASON FOR THE MEETING	

MOUTH AND NOSE PROTECTION ⬤ INDIVIDUAL ⬤ GROUP ⬤

CLOSED ROOM ⬤ OUTDOORS ⬤ CLOSE CONTACT ⬤

CONTACT DETAILS

DATE	PLACE	TIME	REASON FOR THE MEETING	

MOUTH AND NOSE PROTECTION ⬤ INDIVIDUAL ⬤ GROUP ⬤

CLOSED ROOM ⬤ OUTDOORS ⬤ CLOSE CONTACT ⬤

CONTACT DETAILS

DATE	PLACE	TIME	REASON FOR THE MEETING	

MOUTH AND NOSE PROTECTION ⬤ INDIVIDUAL ⬤ GROUP ⬤

CLOSED ROOM ⬤ OUTDOORS ⬤ CLOSE CONTACT ⬤

CONTACT DETAILS

DATE	PLACE	TIME	REASON FOR THE MEETING	

MOUTH AND NOSE PROTECTION ⬤ INDIVIDUAL ⬤ GROUP ⬤

CLOSED ROOM ⬤ OUTDOORS ⬤ CLOSE CONTACT ⬤

CONTACT DETAILS

DATE	PLACE	TIME	REASON FOR THE MEETING	

MOUTH AND NOSE PROTECTION ⬤
CLOSED ROOM ⬤

INDIVIDUAL ⬤
OUTDOORS ⬤

GROUP ⬤
CLOSE CONTACT ⬤

CONTACT DETAILS

DATE	PLACE	TIME	REASON FOR THE MEETING	

MOUTH AND NOSE PROTECTION ⬤
CLOSED ROOM ⬤

INDIVIDUAL ⬤
OUTDOORS ⬤

GROUP ⬤
CLOSE CONTACT ⬤

CONTACT DETAILS

DATE	PLACE	TIME	REASON FOR THE MEETING	

MOUTH AND NOSE PROTECTION ⬤
CLOSED ROOM ⬤

INDIVIDUAL ⬤
OUTDOORS ⬤

GROUP ⬤
CLOSE CONTACT ⬤

CONTACT DETAILS

DATE	PLACE	TIME	REASON FOR THE MEETING	

MOUTH AND NOSE PROTECTION ⬤
CLOSED ROOM ⬤

INDIVIDUAL ⬤
OUTDOORS ⬤

GROUP ⬤
CLOSE CONTACT ⬤

CONTACT DETAILS

DATE	PLACE	TIME		REASON FOR THE MEETING	

MOUTH AND NOSE PROTECTION ◯   INDIVIDUAL ◯   GROUP ◯
CLOSED ROOM ◯   OUTDOORS ◯   CLOSE CONTACT ◯

CONTACT DETAILS

DATE	PLACE	TIME		REASON FOR THE MEETING	

MOUTH AND NOSE PROTECTION ◯   INDIVIDUAL ◯   GROUP ◯
CLOSED ROOM ◯   OUTDOORS ◯   CLOSE CONTACT ◯

CONTACT DETAILS

DATE	PLACE	TIME		REASON FOR THE MEETING	

MOUTH AND NOSE PROTECTION ◯   INDIVIDUAL ◯   GROUP ◯
CLOSED ROOM ◯   OUTDOORS ◯   CLOSE CONTACT ◯

CONTACT DETAILS

DATE	PLACE	TIME		REASON FOR THE MEETING	

MOUTH AND NOSE PROTECTION ◯   INDIVIDUAL ◯   GROUP ◯
CLOSED ROOM ◯   OUTDOORS ◯   CLOSE CONTACT ◯

CONTACT DETAILS

DATE	PLACE	TIME	REASON FOR THE MEETING	

MOUTH AND NOSE PROTECTION ⬤   INDIVIDUAL ⬤   GROUP ⬤
CLOSED ROOM ⬤   OUTDOORS ⬤   CLOSE CONTACT ⬤

CONTACT DETAILS

DATE	PLACE	TIME	REASON FOR THE MEETING	

MOUTH AND NOSE PROTECTION ⬤   INDIVIDUAL ⬤   GROUP ⬤
CLOSED ROOM ⬤   OUTDOORS ⬤   CLOSE CONTACT ⬤

CONTACT DETAILS

DATE	PLACE	TIME	REASON FOR THE MEETING	

MOUTH AND NOSE PROTECTION ⬤   INDIVIDUAL ⬤   GROUP ⬤
CLOSED ROOM ⬤   OUTDOORS ⬤   CLOSE CONTACT ⬤

CONTACT DETAILS

DATE	PLACE	TIME	REASON FOR THE MEETING	

MOUTH AND NOSE PROTECTION ⬤   INDIVIDUAL ⬤   GROUP ⬤
CLOSED ROOM ⬤   OUTDOORS ⬤   CLOSE CONTACT ⬤

CONTACT DETAILS

DATE	PLACE	TIME	REASON FOR THE MEETING	

MOUTH AND NOSE PROTECTION ◯

CLOSED ROOM ◯

INDIVIDUAL ◯ GROUP ◯

OUTDOORS ◯ CLOSE CONTACT ◯

CONTACT DETAILS

DATE	PLACE	TIME	REASON FOR THE MEETING	

MOUTH AND NOSE PROTECTION ◯

CLOSED ROOM ◯

INDIVIDUAL ◯ GROUP ◯

OUTDOORS ◯ CLOSE CONTACT ◯

CONTACT DETAILS

DATE	PLACE	TIME	REASON FOR THE MEETING	

MOUTH AND NOSE PROTECTION ◯

CLOSED ROOM ◯

INDIVIDUAL ◯ GROUP ◯

OUTDOORS ◯ CLOSE CONTACT ◯

CONTACT DETAILS

DATE	PLACE	TIME	REASON FOR THE MEETING	

MOUTH AND NOSE PROTECTION ◯

CLOSED ROOM ◯

INDIVIDUAL ◯ GROUP ◯

OUTDOORS ◯ CLOSE CONTACT ◯

CONTACT DETAILS

DATE	PLACE	TIME	REASON FOR THE MEETING	

MOUTH AND NOSE PROTECTION ◯ INDIVIDUAL ◯ GROUP ◯

CLOSED ROOM ◯ OUTDOORS ◯ CLOSE CONTACT ◯

CONTACT DETAILS

DATE	PLACE	TIME	REASON FOR THE MEETING	

MOUTH AND NOSE PROTECTION ◯ INDIVIDUAL ◯ GROUP ◯

CLOSED ROOM ◯ OUTDOORS ◯ CLOSE CONTACT ◯

CONTACT DETAILS

DATE	PLACE	TIME	REASON FOR THE MEETING	

MOUTH AND NOSE PROTECTION ◯ INDIVIDUAL ◯ GROUP ◯

CLOSED ROOM ◯ OUTDOORS ◯ CLOSE CONTACT ◯

CONTACT DETAILS

DATE	PLACE	TIME	REASON FOR THE MEETING	

MOUTH AND NOSE PROTECTION ◯ INDIVIDUAL ◯ GROUP ◯

CLOSED ROOM ◯ OUTDOORS ◯ CLOSE CONTACT ◯

CONTACT DETAILS

DATE	PLACE	TIME	REASON FOR THE MEETING	

MOUTH AND NOSE PROTECTION ⚪   INDIVIDUAL ⚪   GROUP ⚪

CLOSED ROOM ⚪   OUTDOORS ⚪   CLOSE CONTACT ⚪

CONTACT DETAILS

DATE	PLACE	TIME	REASON FOR THE MEETING	

MOUTH AND NOSE PROTECTION ⚪   INDIVIDUAL ⚪   GROUP ⚪

CLOSED ROOM ⚪   OUTDOORS ⚪   CLOSE CONTACT ⚪

CONTACT DETAILS

DATE	PLACE	TIME	REASON FOR THE MEETING	

MOUTH AND NOSE PROTECTION ⚪   INDIVIDUAL ⚪   GROUP ⚪

CLOSED ROOM ⚪   OUTDOORS ⚪   CLOSE CONTACT ⚪

CONTACT DETAILS

DATE	PLACE	TIME	REASON FOR THE MEETING	

MOUTH AND NOSE PROTECTION ⚪   INDIVIDUAL ⚪   GROUP ⚪

CLOSED ROOM ⚪   OUTDOORS ⚪   CLOSE CONTACT ⚪

CONTACT DETAILS

DATE	PLACE	TIME	REASON FOR THE MEETING	

MOUTH AND NOSE PROTECTION ◯   INDIVIDUAL ◯   GROUP ◯
CLOSED ROOM ◯   OUTDOORS ◯   CLOSE CONTACT ◯

CONTACT DETAILS

DATE	PLACE	TIME	REASON FOR THE MEETING	

MOUTH AND NOSE PROTECTION ◯   INDIVIDUAL ◯   GROUP ◯
CLOSED ROOM ◯   OUTDOORS ◯   CLOSE CONTACT ◯

CONTACT DETAILS

DATE	PLACE	TIME	REASON FOR THE MEETING	

MOUTH AND NOSE PROTECTION ◯   INDIVIDUAL ◯   GROUP ◯
CLOSED ROOM ◯   OUTDOORS ◯   CLOSE CONTACT ◯

CONTACT DETAILS

DATE	PLACE	TIME	REASON FOR THE MEETING	

MOUTH AND NOSE PROTECTION ◯   INDIVIDUAL ◯   GROUP ◯
CLOSED ROOM ◯   OUTDOORS ◯   CLOSE CONTACT ◯

CONTACT DETAILS

DATE	PLACE	TIME	REASON FOR THE MEETING	

MOUTH AND NOSE PROTECTION ● INDIVIDUAL ●   GROUP ●
PROTECTION
CLOSED ROOM ● OUTDOORS ●   CLOSE CONTACT ●

CONTACT DETAILS

DATE	PLACE	TIME	REASON FOR THE MEETING	

MOUTH AND NOSE PROTECTION ● INDIVIDUAL ●   GROUP ●
PROTECTION
CLOSED ROOM ● OUTDOORS ●   CLOSE CONTACT ●

CONTACT DETAILS

DATE	PLACE	TIME	REASON FOR THE MEETING	

MOUTH AND NOSE PROTECTION ● INDIVIDUAL ●   GROUP ●
PROTECTION
CLOSED ROOM ● OUTDOORS ●   CLOSE CONTACT ●

CONTACT DETAILS

DATE	PLACE	TIME	REASON FOR THE MEETING	

MOUTH AND NOSE PROTECTION ● INDIVIDUAL ●   GROUP ●
PROTECTION
CLOSED ROOM ● OUTDOORS ●   CLOSE CONTACT ●

CONTACT DETAILS

DATE	PLACE	TIME	REASON FOR THE MEETING	

MOUTH AND NOSE PROTECTION ⚪
CLOSED ROOM ⚪

INDIVIDUAL ⚪   GROUP ⚪
OUTDOORS ⚪   CLOSE CONTACT ⚪

CONTACT DETAILS

DATE	PLACE	TIME	REASON FOR THE MEETING	

MOUTH AND NOSE PROTECTION ⚪
CLOSED ROOM ⚪

INDIVIDUAL ⚪   GROUP ⚪
OUTDOORS ⚪   CLOSE CONTACT ⚪

CONTACT DETAILS

DATE	PLACE	TIME	REASON FOR THE MEETING	

MOUTH AND NOSE PROTECTION ⚪
CLOSED ROOM ⚪

INDIVIDUAL ⚪   GROUP ⚪
OUTDOORS ⚪   CLOSE CONTACT ⚪

CONTACT DETAILS

DATE	PLACE	TIME	REASON FOR THE MEETING	

MOUTH AND NOSE PROTECTION ⚪
CLOSED ROOM ⚪

INDIVIDUAL ⚪   GROUP ⚪
OUTDOORS ⚪   CLOSE CONTACT ⚪

CONTACT DETAILS

DATE	PLACE	TIME	REASON FOR THE MEETING	

MOUTH AND NOSE PROTECTION ⬤
CLOSED ROOM ⬤

INDIVIDUAL ⬤ GROUP ⬤
OUTDOORS ⬤ CLOSE CONTACT ⬤

CONTACT DETAILS

DATE	PLACE	TIME	REASON FOR THE MEETING	

MOUTH AND NOSE PROTECTION ⬤
CLOSED ROOM ⬤

INDIVIDUAL ⬤ GROUP ⬤
OUTDOORS ⬤ CLOSE CONTACT ⬤

CONTACT DETAILS

DATE	PLACE	TIME	REASON FOR THE MEETING	

MOUTH AND NOSE PROTECTION ⬤
CLOSED ROOM ⬤

INDIVIDUAL ⬤ GROUP ⬤
OUTDOORS ⬤ CLOSE CONTACT ⬤

CONTACT DETAILS

DATE	PLACE	TIME	REASON FOR THE MEETING	

MOUTH AND NOSE PROTECTION ⬤
CLOSED ROOM ⬤

INDIVIDUAL ⬤ GROUP ⬤
OUTDOORS ⬤ CLOSE CONTACT ⬤

CONTACT DETAILS

DATE	PLACE	TIME	REASON FOR THE MEETING	

MOUTH AND NOSE PROTECTION ⬤   INDIVIDUAL ⬤   GROUP ⬤

CLOSED ROOM ⬤   OUTDOORS ⬤   CLOSE CONTACT ⬤

CONTACT DETAILS

DATE	PLACE	TIME	REASON FOR THE MEETING	

MOUTH AND NOSE PROTECTION ⬤   INDIVIDUAL ⬤   GROUP ⬤

CLOSED ROOM ⬤   OUTDOORS ⬤   CLOSE CONTACT ⬤

CONTACT DETAILS

DATE	PLACE	TIME	REASON FOR THE MEETING	

MOUTH AND NOSE PROTECTION ⬤   INDIVIDUAL ⬤   GROUP ⬤

CLOSED ROOM ⬤   OUTDOORS ⬤   CLOSE CONTACT ⬤

CONTACT DETAILS

DATE	PLACE	TIME	REASON FOR THE MEETING	

MOUTH AND NOSE PROTECTION ⬤   INDIVIDUAL ⬤   GROUP ⬤

CLOSED ROOM ⬤   OUTDOORS ⬤   CLOSE CONTACT ⬤

CONTACT DETAILS

DATE	PLACE	TIME	REASON FOR THE MEETING	

MOUTH AND NOSE PROTECTION ⬤   INDIVIDUAL ⬤   GROUP ⬤

CLOSED ROOM ⬤   OUTDOORS ⬤   CLOSE CONTACT ⬤

CONTACT DETAILS

DATE	PLACE	TIME	REASON FOR THE MEETING	

MOUTH AND NOSE PROTECTION ⬤   INDIVIDUAL ⬤   GROUP ⬤

CLOSED ROOM ⬤   OUTDOORS ⬤   CLOSE CONTACT ⬤

CONTACT DETAILS

DATE	PLACE	TIME	REASON FOR THE MEETING	

MOUTH AND NOSE PROTECTION ⬤   INDIVIDUAL ⬤   GROUP ⬤

CLOSED ROOM ⬤   OUTDOORS ⬤   CLOSE CONTACT ⬤

CONTACT DETAILS

DATE	PLACE	TIME	REASON FOR THE MEETING	

MOUTH AND NOSE PROTECTION ⬤   INDIVIDUAL ⬤   GROUP ⬤

CLOSED ROOM ⬤   OUTDOORS ⬤   CLOSE CONTACT ⬤

CONTACT DETAILS

DATE	PLACE	TIME	REASON FOR THE MEETING	

MOUTH AND NOSE PROTECTION ⬤
CLOSED ROOM ⬤
INDIVIDUAL ⬤
OUTDOORS ⬤
GROUP ⬤
CLOSE CONTACT ⬤

CONTACT DETAILS

DATE	PLACE	TIME	REASON FOR THE MEETING	

MOUTH AND NOSE PROTECTION ⬤
CLOSED ROOM ⬤
INDIVIDUAL ⬤
OUTDOORS ⬤
GROUP ⬤
CLOSE CONTACT ⬤

CONTACT DETAILS

DATE	PLACE	TIME	REASON FOR THE MEETING	

MOUTH AND NOSE PROTECTION ⬤
CLOSED ROOM ⬤
INDIVIDUAL ⬤
OUTDOORS ⬤
GROUP ⬤
CLOSE CONTACT ⬤

CONTACT DETAILS

DATE	PLACE	TIME	REASON FOR THE MEETING	

MOUTH AND NOSE PROTECTION ⬤
CLOSED ROOM ⬤
INDIVIDUAL ⬤
OUTDOORS ⬤
GROUP ⬤
CLOSE CONTACT ⬤

CONTACT DETAILS

DATE	PLACE	TIME	REASON FOR THE MEETING	

MOUTH AND NOSE PROTECTION ⬤   INDIVIDUAL ⬤   GROUP ⬤
CLOSED ROOM ⬤   OUTDOORS ⬤   CLOSE CONTACT ⬤

CONTACT DETAILS

DATE	PLACE	TIME	REASON FOR THE MEETING	

MOUTH AND NOSE PROTECTION ⬤   INDIVIDUAL ⬤   GROUP ⬤
CLOSED ROOM ⬤   OUTDOORS ⬤   CLOSE CONTACT ⬤

CONTACT DETAILS

DATE	PLACE	TIME	REASON FOR THE MEETING	

MOUTH AND NOSE PROTECTION ⬤   INDIVIDUAL ⬤   GROUP ⬤
CLOSED ROOM ⬤   OUTDOORS ⬤   CLOSE CONTACT ⬤

CONTACT DETAILS

DATE	PLACE	TIME	REASON FOR THE MEETING	

MOUTH AND NOSE PROTECTION ⬤   INDIVIDUAL ⬤   GROUP ⬤
CLOSED ROOM ⬤   OUTDOORS ⬤   CLOSE CONTACT ⬤

CONTACT DETAILS

DATE	PLACE	TIME		REASON FOR THE MEETING	

| MOUTH AND NOSE PROTECTION ○ | | INDIVIDUAL ○ | GROUP ○ |
| CLOSED ROOM ○ | | OUTDOORS ○ | CLOSE CONTACT ○ |

CONTACT DETAILS

DATE	PLACE	TIME		REASON FOR THE MEETING	

| MOUTH AND NOSE PROTECTION ○ | | INDIVIDUAL ○ | GROUP ○ |
| CLOSED ROOM ○ | | OUTDOORS ○ | CLOSE CONTACT ○ |

CONTACT DETAILS

DATE	PLACE	TIME		REASON FOR THE MEETING	

| MOUTH AND NOSE PROTECTION ○ | | INDIVIDUAL ○ | GROUP ○ |
| CLOSED ROOM ○ | | OUTDOORS ○ | CLOSE CONTACT ○ |

CONTACT DETAILS

DATE	PLACE	TIME		REASON FOR THE MEETING	

| MOUTH AND NOSE PROTECTION ○ | | INDIVIDUAL ○ | GROUP ○ |
| CLOSED ROOM ○ | | OUTDOORS ○ | CLOSE CONTACT ○ |

CONTACT DETAILS

DATE	PLACE	TIME	REASON FOR THE MEETING	

MOUTH AND NOSE PROTECTION ⬤   INDIVIDUAL ⬤   GROUP ⬤
CLOSED ROOM ⬤   OUTDOORS ⬤   CLOSE CONTACT ⬤

CONTACT DETAILS

DATE	PLACE	TIME	REASON FOR THE MEETING	

MOUTH AND NOSE PROTECTION ⬤   INDIVIDUAL ⬤   GROUP ⬤
CLOSED ROOM ⬤   OUTDOORS ⬤   CLOSE CONTACT ⬤

CONTACT DETAILS

DATE	PLACE	TIME	REASON FOR THE MEETING	

MOUTH AND NOSE PROTECTION ⬤   INDIVIDUAL ⬤   GROUP ⬤
CLOSED ROOM ⬤   OUTDOORS ⬤   CLOSE CONTACT ⬤

CONTACT DETAILS

DATE	PLACE	TIME	REASON FOR THE MEETING	

MOUTH AND NOSE PROTECTION ⬤   INDIVIDUAL ⬤   GROUP ⬤
CLOSED ROOM ⬤   OUTDOORS ⬤   CLOSE CONTACT ⬤

CONTACT DETAILS

DATE	PLACE	TIME	REASON FOR THE MEETING	

MOUTH AND NOSE PROTECTION ⚪
CLOSED ROOM ⚪
INDIVIDUAL ⚪ GROUP ⚪
OUTDOORS ⚪ CLOSE CONTACT ⚪

CONTACT DETAILS

DATE	PLACE	TIME	REASON FOR THE MEETING	

MOUTH AND NOSE PROTECTION ⚪
CLOSED ROOM ⚪
INDIVIDUAL ⚪ GROUP ⚪
OUTDOORS ⚪ CLOSE CONTACT ⚪

CONTACT DETAILS

DATE	PLACE	TIME	REASON FOR THE MEETING	

MOUTH AND NOSE PROTECTION ⚪
CLOSED ROOM ⚪
INDIVIDUAL ⚪ GROUP ⚪
OUTDOORS ⚪ CLOSE CONTACT ⚪

CONTACT DETAILS

DATE	PLACE	TIME	REASON FOR THE MEETING	

MOUTH AND NOSE PROTECTION ⚪
CLOSED ROOM ⚪
INDIVIDUAL ⚪ GROUP ⚪
OUTDOORS ⚪ CLOSE CONTACT ⚪

CONTACT DETAILS

DATE	PLACE	TIME	REASON FOR THE MEETING	

MOUTH AND NOSE PROTECTION ⚪
CLOSED ROOM ⚪

INDIVIDUAL ⚪   GROUP ⚪
OUTDOORS ⚪   CLOSE CONTACT ⚪

CONTACT DETAILS

DATE	PLACE	TIME	REASON FOR THE MEETING	

MOUTH AND NOSE PROTECTION ⚪
CLOSED ROOM ⚪

INDIVIDUAL ⚪   GROUP ⚪
OUTDOORS ⚪   CLOSE CONTACT ⚪

CONTACT DETAILS

DATE	PLACE	TIME	REASON FOR THE MEETING	

MOUTH AND NOSE PROTECTION ⚪
CLOSED ROOM ⚪

INDIVIDUAL ⚪   GROUP ⚪
OUTDOORS ⚪   CLOSE CONTACT ⚪

CONTACT DETAILS

DATE	PLACE	TIME	REASON FOR THE MEETING	

MOUTH AND NOSE PROTECTION ⚪
CLOSED ROOM ⚪

INDIVIDUAL ⚪   GROUP ⚪
OUTDOORS ⚪   CLOSE CONTACT ⚪

CONTACT DETAILS

DATE	PLACE	TIME	REASON FOR THE MEETING	

MOUTH AND NOSE PROTECTION ⚪ INDIVIDUAL ⚪ GROUP ⚪
CLOSED ROOM ⚪ OUTDOORS ⚪ CLOSE CONTACT ⚪

CONTACT DETAILS

DATE	PLACE	TIME	REASON FOR THE MEETING	

MOUTH AND NOSE PROTECTION ⚪ INDIVIDUAL ⚪ GROUP ⚪
CLOSED ROOM ⚪ OUTDOORS ⚪ CLOSE CONTACT ⚪

CONTACT DETAILS

DATE	PLACE	TIME	REASON FOR THE MEETING	

MOUTH AND NOSE PROTECTION ⚪ INDIVIDUAL ⚪ GROUP ⚪
CLOSED ROOM ⚪ OUTDOORS ⚪ CLOSE CONTACT ⚪

CONTACT DETAILS

DATE	PLACE	TIME	REASON FOR THE MEETING	

MOUTH AND NOSE PROTECTION ⚪ INDIVIDUAL ⚪ GROUP ⚪
CLOSED ROOM ⚪ OUTDOORS ⚪ CLOSE CONTACT ⚪

CONTACT DETAILS

DATE	PLACE	TIME	REASON FOR THE MEETING	

MOUTH AND NOSE PROTECTION ⬤   INDIVIDUAL ⬤   GROUP ⬤
CLOSED ROOM ⬤   OUTDOORS ⬤   CLOSE CONTACT ⬤

CONTACT DETAILS

DATE	PLACE	TIME	REASON FOR THE MEETING	

MOUTH AND NOSE PROTECTION ⬤   INDIVIDUAL ⬤   GROUP ⬤
CLOSED ROOM ⬤   OUTDOORS ⬤   CLOSE CONTACT ⬤

CONTACT DETAILS

DATE	PLACE	TIME	REASON FOR THE MEETING	

MOUTH AND NOSE PROTECTION ⬤   INDIVIDUAL ⬤   GROUP ⬤
CLOSED ROOM ⬤   OUTDOORS ⬤   CLOSE CONTACT ⬤

CONTACT DETAILS

DATE	PLACE	TIME	REASON FOR THE MEETING	

MOUTH AND NOSE PROTECTION ⬤   INDIVIDUAL ⬤   GROUP ⬤
CLOSED ROOM ⬤   OUTDOORS ⬤   CLOSE CONTACT ⬤

CONTACT DETAILS

DATE	PLACE	TIME	REASON FOR THE MEETING	

MOUTH AND NOSE PROTECTION ⬤   INDIVIDUAL ⬤   GROUP ⬤
CLOSED ROOM ⬤   OUTDOORS ⬤   CLOSE CONTACT ⬤

CONTACT DETAILS

DATE	PLACE	TIME	REASON FOR THE MEETING	

MOUTH AND NOSE PROTECTION ⬤   INDIVIDUAL ⬤   GROUP ⬤
CLOSED ROOM ⬤   OUTDOORS ⬤   CLOSE CONTACT ⬤

CONTACT DETAILS

DATE	PLACE	TIME	REASON FOR THE MEETING	

MOUTH AND NOSE PROTECTION ⬤   INDIVIDUAL ⬤   GROUP ⬤
CLOSED ROOM ⬤   OUTDOORS ⬤   CLOSE CONTACT ⬤

CONTACT DETAILS

DATE	PLACE	TIME	REASON FOR THE MEETING	

MOUTH AND NOSE PROTECTION ⬤   INDIVIDUAL ⬤   GROUP ⬤
CLOSED ROOM ⬤   OUTDOORS ⬤   CLOSE CONTACT ⬤

CONTACT DETAILS

DATE	PLACE	TIME	REASON FOR THE MEETING	

	MOUTH AND NOSE PROTECTION ⬤	INDIVIDUAL ⬤	GROUP ⬤
	CLOSED ROOM ⬤	OUTDOORS ⬤	CLOSE CONTACT ⬤

CONTACT DETAILS

DATE	PLACE	TIME	REASON FOR THE MEETING	

	MOUTH AND NOSE PROTECTION ⬤	INDIVIDUAL ⬤	GROUP ⬤
	CLOSED ROOM ⬤	OUTDOORS ⬤	CLOSE CONTACT ⬤

CONTACT DETAILS

DATE	PLACE	TIME	REASON FOR THE MEETING	

	MOUTH AND NOSE PROTECTION ⬤	INDIVIDUAL ⬤	GROUP ⬤
	CLOSED ROOM ⬤	OUTDOORS ⬤	CLOSE CONTACT ⬤

CONTACT DETAILS

DATE	PLACE	TIME	REASON FOR THE MEETING	

	MOUTH AND NOSE PROTECTION ⬤	INDIVIDUAL ⬤	GROUP ⬤
	CLOSED ROOM ⬤	OUTDOORS ⬤	CLOSE CONTACT ⬤

CONTACT DETAILS

DATE	PLACE	TIME	REASON FOR THE MEETING	

MOUTH AND NOSE PROTECTION ●   INDIVIDUAL ●   GROUP ●

CLOSED ROOM ●   OUTDOORS ●   CLOSE CONTACT ●

CONTACT DETAILS

DATE	PLACE	TIME	REASON FOR THE MEETING	

MOUTH AND NOSE PROTECTION ●   INDIVIDUAL ●   GROUP ●

CLOSED ROOM ●   OUTDOORS ●   CLOSE CONTACT ●

CONTACT DETAILS

DATE	PLACE	TIME	REASON FOR THE MEETING	

MOUTH AND NOSE PROTECTION ●   INDIVIDUAL ●   GROUP ●

CLOSED ROOM ●   OUTDOORS ●   CLOSE CONTACT ●

CONTACT DETAILS

DATE	PLACE	TIME	REASON FOR THE MEETING	

MOUTH AND NOSE PROTECTION ●   INDIVIDUAL ●   GROUP ●

CLOSED ROOM ●   OUTDOORS ●   CLOSE CONTACT ●

CONTACT DETAILS

DATE	PLACE	TIME	REASON FOR THE MEETING	

MOUTH AND NOSE PROTECTION ⬤   INDIVIDUAL ⬤   GROUP ⬤

CLOSED ROOM ⬤   OUTDOORS ⬤   CLOSE CONTACT ⬤

CONTACT DETAILS

DATE	PLACE	TIME	REASON FOR THE MEETING	

MOUTH AND NOSE PROTECTION ⬤   INDIVIDUAL ⬤   GROUP ⬤

CLOSED ROOM ⬤   OUTDOORS ⬤   CLOSE CONTACT ⬤

CONTACT DETAILS

DATE	PLACE	TIME	REASON FOR THE MEETING	

MOUTH AND NOSE PROTECTION ⬤   INDIVIDUAL ⬤   GROUP ⬤

CLOSED ROOM ⬤   OUTDOORS ⬤   CLOSE CONTACT ⬤

CONTACT DETAILS

DATE	PLACE	TIME	REASON FOR THE MEETING	

MOUTH AND NOSE PROTECTION ⬤   INDIVIDUAL ⬤   GROUP ⬤

CLOSED ROOM ⬤   OUTDOORS ⬤   CLOSE CONTACT ⬤

CONTACT DETAILS

DATE	PLACE	TIME	REASON FOR THE MEETING	

MOUTH AND NOSE PROTECTION ⚪
CLOSED ROOM ⚪

INDIVIDUAL ⚪   GROUP ⚪
OUTDOORS ⚪   CLOSE CONTACT ⚪

CONTACT DETAILS

DATE	PLACE	TIME	REASON FOR THE MEETING	

MOUTH AND NOSE PROTECTION ⚪
CLOSED ROOM ⚪

INDIVIDUAL ⚪   GROUP ⚪
OUTDOORS ⚪   CLOSE CONTACT ⚪

CONTACT DETAILS

DATE	PLACE	TIME	REASON FOR THE MEETING	

MOUTH AND NOSE PROTECTION ⚪
CLOSED ROOM ⚪

INDIVIDUAL ⚪   GROUP ⚪
OUTDOORS ⚪   CLOSE CONTACT ⚪

CONTACT DETAILS

DATE	PLACE	TIME	REASON FOR THE MEETING	

MOUTH AND NOSE PROTECTION ⚪
CLOSED ROOM ⚪

INDIVIDUAL ⚪   GROUP ⚪
OUTDOORS ⚪   CLOSE CONTACT ⚪

CONTACT DETAILS

DATE	PLACE	TIME		REASON FOR THE MEETING	

MOUTH AND NOSE PROTECTION ⚪
CLOSED ROOM ⚪

INDIVIDUAL ⚪   GROUP ⚪
OUTDOORS ⚪   CLOSE CONTACT ⚪

CONTACT DETAILS

DATE	PLACE	TIME		REASON FOR THE MEETING	

MOUTH AND NOSE PROTECTION ⚪
CLOSED ROOM ⚪

INDIVIDUAL ⚪   GROUP ⚪
OUTDOORS ⚪   CLOSE CONTACT ⚪

CONTACT DETAILS

DATE	PLACE	TIME		REASON FOR THE MEETING	

MOUTH AND NOSE PROTECTION ⚪
CLOSED ROOM ⚪

INDIVIDUAL ⚪   GROUP ⚪
OUTDOORS ⚪   CLOSE CONTACT ⚪

CONTACT DETAILS

DATE	PLACE	TIME		REASON FOR THE MEETING	

MOUTH AND NOSE PROTECTION ⚪
CLOSED ROOM ⚪

INDIVIDUAL ⚪   GROUP ⚪
OUTDOORS ⚪   CLOSE CONTACT ⚪

CONTACT DETAILS

DATE	PLACE	TIME	REASON FOR THE MEETING	

MOUTH AND NOSE PROTECTION ⬤   INDIVIDUAL ⬤   GROUP ⬤

CLOSED ROOM ⬤   OUTDOORS ⬤   CLOSE CONTACT ⬤

CONTACT DETAILS

DATE	PLACE	TIME	REASON FOR THE MEETING	

MOUTH AND NOSE PROTECTION ⬤   INDIVIDUAL ⬤   GROUP ⬤

CLOSED ROOM ⬤   OUTDOORS ⬤   CLOSE CONTACT ⬤

CONTACT DETAILS

DATE	PLACE	TIME	REASON FOR THE MEETING	

MOUTH AND NOSE PROTECTION ⬤   INDIVIDUAL ⬤   GROUP ⬤

CLOSED ROOM ⬤   OUTDOORS ⬤   CLOSE CONTACT ⬤

CONTACT DETAILS

DATE	PLACE	TIME	REASON FOR THE MEETING	

MOUTH AND NOSE PROTECTION ⬤   INDIVIDUAL ⬤   GROUP ⬤

CLOSED ROOM ⬤   OUTDOORS ⬤   CLOSE CONTACT ⬤

CONTACT DETAILS

DATE	PLACE	TIME	REASON FOR THE MEETING	

MOUTH AND NOSE PROTECTION ⚪   INDIVIDUAL ⚪   GROUP ⚪

CLOSED ROOM ⚪   OUTDOORS ⚪   CLOSE CONTACT ⚪

CONTACT DETAILS

DATE	PLACE	TIME	REASON FOR THE MEETING	

MOUTH AND NOSE PROTECTION ⚪   INDIVIDUAL ⚪   GROUP ⚪

CLOSED ROOM ⚪   OUTDOORS ⚪   CLOSE CONTACT ⚪

CONTACT DETAILS

DATE	PLACE	TIME	REASON FOR THE MEETING	

MOUTH AND NOSE PROTECTION ⚪   INDIVIDUAL ⚪   GROUP ⚪

CLOSED ROOM ⚪   OUTDOORS ⚪   CLOSE CONTACT ⚪

CONTACT DETAILS

DATE	PLACE	TIME	REASON FOR THE MEETING	

MOUTH AND NOSE PROTECTION ⚪   INDIVIDUAL ⚪   GROUP ⚪

CLOSED ROOM ⚪   OUTDOORS ⚪   CLOSE CONTACT ⚪

CONTACT DETAILS

DATE	PLACE	TIME	REASON FOR THE MEETING	

MOUTH AND NOSE PROTECTION ⚪
PROTECTION
CLOSED ROOM ⚪

INDIVIDUAL ⚪   GROUP ⚪
OUTDOORS ⚪   CLOSE CONTACT ⚪

CONTACT DETAILS

DATE	PLACE	TIME	REASON FOR THE MEETING	

MOUTH AND NOSE PROTECTION ⚪
CLOSED ROOM ⚪

INDIVIDUAL ⚪   GROUP ⚪
OUTDOORS ⚪   CLOSE CONTACT ⚪

CONTACT DETAILS

DATE	PLACE	TIME	REASON FOR THE MEETING	

MOUTH AND NOSE PROTECTION ⚪
CLOSED ROOM ⚪

INDIVIDUAL ⚪   GROUP ⚪
OUTDOORS ⚪   CLOSE CONTACT ⚪

CONTACT DETAILS

DATE	PLACE	TIME	REASON FOR THE MEETING	

MOUTH AND NOSE PROTECTION ⚪
CLOSED ROOM ⚪

INDIVIDUAL ⚪   GROUP ⚪
OUTDOORS ⚪   CLOSE CONTACT ⚪

CONTACT DETAILS

DATE	PLACE	TIME	REASON FOR THE MEETING	

MOUTH AND NOSE PROTECTION ⚪
CLOSED ROOM ⚪

INDIVIDUAL ⚪
OUTDOORS ⚪

GROUP ⚪
CLOSE CONTACT ⚪

CONTACT DETAILS

DATE	PLACE	TIME	REASON FOR THE MEETING	

MOUTH AND NOSE PROTECTION ⚪
CLOSED ROOM ⚪

INDIVIDUAL ⚪
OUTDOORS ⚪

GROUP ⚪
CLOSE CONTACT ⚪

CONTACT DETAILS

DATE	PLACE	TIME	REASON FOR THE MEETING	

MOUTH AND NOSE PROTECTION ⚪
CLOSED ROOM ⚪

INDIVIDUAL ⚪
OUTDOORS ⚪

GROUP ⚪
CLOSE CONTACT ⚪

CONTACT DETAILS

DATE	PLACE	TIME	REASON FOR THE MEETING	

MOUTH AND NOSE PROTECTION ⚪
CLOSED ROOM ⚪

INDIVIDUAL ⚪
OUTDOORS ⚪

GROUP ⚪
CLOSE CONTACT ⚪

CONTACT DETAILS

DATE	PLACE	TIME	REASON FOR THE MEETING	

MOUTH AND NOSE PROTECTION ⬤   INDIVIDUAL ⬤   GROUP ⬤

CLOSED ROOM ⬤   OUTDOORS ⬤   CLOSE CONTACT ⬤

CONTACT DETAILS

DATE	PLACE	TIME	REASON FOR THE MEETING	

MOUTH AND NOSE PROTECTION ⬤   INDIVIDUAL ⬤   GROUP ⬤

CLOSED ROOM ⬤   OUTDOORS ⬤   CLOSE CONTACT ⬤

CONTACT DETAILS

DATE	PLACE	TIME	REASON FOR THE MEETING	

MOUTH AND NOSE PROTECTION ⬤   INDIVIDUAL ⬤   GROUP ⬤

CLOSED ROOM ⬤   OUTDOORS ⬤   CLOSE CONTACT ⬤

CONTACT DETAILS

DATE	PLACE	TIME	REASON FOR THE MEETING	

MOUTH AND NOSE PROTECTION ⬤   INDIVIDUAL ⬤   GROUP ⬤

CLOSED ROOM ⬤   OUTDOORS ⬤   CLOSE CONTACT ⬤

CONTACT DETAILS

DATE	PLACE	TIME	REASON FOR THE MEETING	

MOUTH AND NOSE PROTECTION ⬤ INDIVIDUAL ⬤ GROUP ⬤

CLOSED ROOM ⬤ OUTDOORS ⬤ CLOSE CONTACT ⬤

CONTACT DETAILS

DATE	PLACE	TIME	REASON FOR THE MEETING	

MOUTH AND NOSE PROTECTION ⬤ INDIVIDUAL ⬤ GROUP ⬤

CLOSED ROOM ⬤ OUTDOORS ⬤ CLOSE CONTACT ⬤

CONTACT DETAILS

DATE	PLACE	TIME	REASON FOR THE MEETING	

MOUTH AND NOSE PROTECTION ⬤ INDIVIDUAL ⬤ GROUP ⬤

CLOSED ROOM ⬤ OUTDOORS ⬤ CLOSE CONTACT ⬤

CONTACT DETAILS

DATE	PLACE	TIME	REASON FOR THE MEETING	

MOUTH AND NOSE PROTECTION ⬤ INDIVIDUAL ⬤ GROUP ⬤

CLOSED ROOM ⬤ OUTDOORS ⬤ CLOSE CONTACT ⬤

CONTACT DETAILS

DATE	PLACE	TIME	REASON FOR THE MEETING	

MOUTH AND NOSE PROTECTION ⚪   INDIVIDUAL ⚪   GROUP ⚪
CLOSED ROOM ⚪   OUTDOORS ⚪   CLOSE CONTACT ⚪

CONTACT DETAILS

DATE	PLACE	TIME	REASON FOR THE MEETING	

MOUTH AND NOSE PROTECTION ⚪   INDIVIDUAL ⚪   GROUP ⚪
CLOSED ROOM ⚪   OUTDOORS ⚪   CLOSE CONTACT ⚪

CONTACT DETAILS

DATE	PLACE	TIME	REASON FOR THE MEETING	

MOUTH AND NOSE PROTECTION ⚪   INDIVIDUAL ⚪   GROUP ⚪
CLOSED ROOM ⚪   OUTDOORS ⚪   CLOSE CONTACT ⚪

CONTACT DETAILS

DATE	PLACE	TIME	REASON FOR THE MEETING	

MOUTH AND NOSE PROTECTION ⚪   INDIVIDUAL ⚪   GROUP ⚪
CLOSED ROOM ⚪   OUTDOORS ⚪   CLOSE CONTACT ⚪

CONTACT DETAILS

DATE	PLACE	TIME	REASON FOR THE MEETING	

	MOUTH AND NOSE PROTECTION ⬤		INDIVIDUAL ⬤	GROUP ⬤
	CLOSED ROOM ⬤		OUTDOORS ⬤	CLOSE CONTACT ⬤

CONTACT DETAILS

DATE	PLACE	TIME	REASON FOR THE MEETING	

	MOUTH AND NOSE PROTECTION ⬤		INDIVIDUAL ⬤	GROUP ⬤
	CLOSED ROOM ⬤		OUTDOORS ⬤	CLOSE CONTACT ⬤

CONTACT DETAILS

DATE	PLACE	TIME	REASON FOR THE MEETING	

	MOUTH AND NOSE PROTECTION ⬤		INDIVIDUAL ⬤	GROUP ⬤
	CLOSED ROOM ⬤		OUTDOORS ⬤	CLOSE CONTACT ⬤

CONTACT DETAILS

DATE	PLACE	TIME	REASON FOR THE MEETING	

	MOUTH AND NOSE PROTECTION ⬤		INDIVIDUAL ⬤	GROUP ⬤
	CLOSED ROOM ⬤		OUTDOORS ⬤	CLOSE CONTACT ⬤

CONTACT DETAILS